# The Art of Mindfulness for Fitness and Nutritional Balance

# Table of Contents

# Chapter 1. Introduction

In the bustling whirlwind of modern life, paying attention to one's health - both physically and nutritionally - can often take a back burner. However, here's an invigorating twist - our Special Report titled "The Art of Mindfulness for Fitness and Nutritional Balance." This report embodies not just the practical know-hows, but an exciting blend of mindfulness methods and how to infuse it in your fitness and nutritional regimes. Aimed to guide you towards a healthier version of yourself, this report resonates with vibrant energy and promises a journey that's as nourishing as it is enlightening. Whether you're a fitness enthusiast, a nutrition fanatic, or someone simply seeking balance in their life, this report is just the companion you need. As you navigate through our meticulously curated content, prepare to renew your perspective, and reignite your relationship with health and wellbeing. Strap in and let's journey together towards a more mindful, fit, and nutritiously balanced lifestyle!

# Chapter 2. The Intersection of Mindfulness, Fitness, and Nutrition

The path to achieving a harmonious blend of mindfulness, fitness, and nutrition can seem elusive. However, learning how to intertwine these aspects can greatly enhance overall wellbeing. This journey starts by understanding mindfulness - being fully aware and present in each moment, avoiding judgmental thoughts or overreacting to situations.

## 2.1. Understanding Mindfulness

Mindfulness is primarily about being present in the moment and paying close attention to one's feelings, thoughts, and sensations in a non-judgmental way. It's about cultivating awareness and acceptance of your experiences, emotions, and thoughts.

The practice of mindfulness means being fully engaged in whatever activity you're doing, whether it's eating a meal, exercising, or simply just breathing. This sense of presence and engagement enables a more profound and nuanced understanding of various life experiences, leading to increased well-being and fulfilment.

Incorporating mindfulness into your fitness and nutrition regime can be a transformative decision. The key is to listen to your body, respect its signals, and respond effectively.

## 2.2. The Role of Mindfulness in Fitness

Now let's delve into the realm of fitness. Introducing mindfulness into your exercises might elevate your workouts to a whole new level. It encourages focus, boosts motivation, and pushes you to listen to your body more attentively.

Making your workouts mindful means paying undivided attention to the way your body moves during each exercise, the rhythm of your breath, your heart rate, and even the sensations that course through your muscles. It's about learning to distinguish between healthy discomfort and pain that signifies injury. This deliberate focus can help in improving form, preventing injuries, and enhancing your overall fitness experience.

## 2.3. Mindful Nutrition

Food is not just fuel for the body; it also impacts our emotions and mental health. Mindful eating is a process in which we bring our attention to the experience of eating, savoring each bite, and relishing the flavors, textures, and smells.

This practice helps us better appreciate food, prevents overeating, promotes better digestion, and allows us to identify our body's hunger and satiety cues more clearly. In such a way, we can make healthier food choices and develop a more balanced and respectful relationship with food.

## 2.4. Fusion of Mindfulness, Fitness, and Nutrition

When mindfulness, fitness, and nutrition come together, it leads to an enhanced state of physical, emotional, and psychological wellbeing.

In a fitness regimen, mindfulness prompts commitment, precision, flexibility, and, most importantly, listening to your body. On the other hand, in the nutrition realm, it persuades sensible eating, discerning hunger and satisfaction cues, and recognizing the emotional connections with food.

The combination of mindful fitness and nutrition becomes a powerful tool for transformation. It changes the way you view your fitness routine and dietary habits. It can make you more conscious of your body, lead you to make healthier choices, and achieve your fitness goals more efficiently.

## 2.5. Techniques to Implement Mindfulness

1. Breathing Techniques: Concentration on breath teaches you to concentrate on one task at a time, fostering mindfulness.

2. Mindful Eating Practises: Pay heed to what you consume. Take time to taste and enjoy every bite.

3. Mindful Exercise: Be conscious of your bodily movements, understand your body, and respect its limits.

4. Daily Meditation: It helps clear your mind and encourage focus.

Applying these techniques can help you integrate mindfulness into your fitness and nutrition regimen.

# 2.6. The Benefits of Integrating Mindfulness

The integration of mindfulness with fitness and nutrition comes with several benefits:

1. Greater Appreciation of Food: Mindful eating lets you appreciate the flavors, textures, and colors of your food.

2. Improved Digestion and Nutrient Absorption: Eating slowly and chewing thoroughly can improve digestion and allow better nutrient absorption.

3. Enhanced Exercise Performance: Mindful exercise leads to better form and enhanced performance.

4. Reduced Risk of Overeating: Being more aware of your hunger and fullness cues can help prevent overeating.

5. Lower Stress Levels: Mindful practices such as meditation can help manage stress levels.

In conclusion, embracing the coalescence of mindfulness, fitness, and nutrition could usher in profound changes in your lifestyle. It's not just about achieving physical goals, but more about establishing a vigorous connection with yourself, allowing self-growth, and making room for enriched life experiences. Much like a journey, it takes time and effort to master, but the long-term benefits on the mind, body, and soul are entirely worth it.

# Chapter 3. Understanding the Role of Mindfulness in Wellness

Mindfulness is a powerful practice that, when embraced, can significantly enhance overall wellness by fostering an acute awareness of our physical and emotional state. It can teach us to consciously pay attention to our bodies, understand our feelings, desires, and needs, hence, allowing us to make healthier choices for ourselves. As research indicates, this can lead to improvements in physical, mental, and emotional health.

## 3.1. The Concept of Mindfulness

Mindfulness refers to the practice of focusing attention on the present moment and accepting it without judgment. Jon Kabat-Zinn, a renowned mindfulness researcher, and practitioner, often describes mindfulness as "paying attention in a particular way, on purpose, in the present moment, non-judgmentally."

The wellspring of mindfulness is meditation, an ancient practice found in a broad range of spiritual and philosophical traditions. However, it's essential to remember that mindfulness is not solely a religious practice, but rather a set of techniques to cultivate awareness and focus, that can be applied and utilized by anyone.

## 3.2. Mindfulness and the Mind-Body Connection

The mind-body connection refers to the relationship between our thoughts, feelings, social interactions, and overall health. In recent years, the understanding of this connection has expanded significantly. One essential aspect of the mind-body connection is how our mind influences our physical health.

Mindfulness helps strengthen the mind-body connection by making us more aware of the sensations in our bodies and redirecting our focus towards them. By doing this, we are not only drawn away from harmful negative thoughts and stressors but are also better able to listen to our body's needs.

## 3.3. Mindfulness in Everyday Activities

By consciously focusing on the minute details of our everyday activities, we can practice mindfulness. Whether it's savoring the taste of your tea, focusing on your breathing, or simply feeling the texture of the clothes you're wearing, each of these actions serves as an opportunity to anchor your mind in the present.

Here's an exercise: next time you're eating a meal, bring your entire mindfulness to the food. Notice its color, shape, and aroma. As you take a bite, pay attention to the texture and the flavor that floods your mouth. Recognizing each aspect of this seemingly mundane task allows you to practice mindfulness and helps you connect deeper with your self and your experience.

## 3.4. Mindfulness and Physical Health

Mindfulness has been associated with numerous physical health benefits. By helping reduce stress and anxiety, it can indirectly lead to lowering blood pressure and heart rate, improving sleep, and even increasing pain tolerance. Greater mindfulness can also improve our physical fitness by enhancing our exercise experiences and allowing us to be more in tune with our body's needs and capabilities during physical exertion.

One study published in the Journal of Health Psychology found that individuals who practice mindfulness regularly have a lower body mass index (BMI), indicating a healthier body weight and less risk of obesity. Furthermore, mindfulness can also aid in healthier eating choices and practices, often referred to as mindful eating.

## 3.5. Mindfulness and Mental Health

Just as there are physical health benefits, mindfulness plays a critical role in mental and emotional wellbeing. Studies show that mindfulness can help manage depression, anxiety, and post-traumatic stress disorder (PTSD). Through regular practice, mindfulness can reduce the brain's tendency to fall into detrimental patterns of overthinking, catastrophizing, or persistently focusing on negative aspects of ourselves or our lives.

Additionally, by fostering a state of intentional awareness, mindfulness can help us better differentiate between constructive and destructive emotions, aiding in emotional regulation. It teaches us to respond to our feelings, rather than reacting impulsively, promoting healthy emotional processing and expression.

## 3.6. Incorporating Mindfulness Into Your Lifestyle

Incorporating mindfulness into your daily routine might seem challenging at first, as it does demand a shift in the way you interact with your day-to-day experiences. However, starting with small steps can make it more manageable. Try to dedicate a few minutes each day to sit in silence, focusing on your breathing. Practice mindful eating during one meal each day, paying attention to the scents, tastes, and textures of your food.

Also, consider trying a mindfulness-based technique such as yoga or tai chi, which integrate physical movement with mindfulness practice. These activities can help you learn to focus on how different parts of your body feel and move.

Overall, introducing mindfulness into your life is a journey that requires one step at a time, but the rewards in terms of improved wellness are profound and well worth the effort.

In conclusion, mindfulness serves as a tool for us to perceive the world in a more direct, clear manner, deepening our understanding and appreciation for life. Its effect on wellness underscores the importance of being present in the here and now, teaching us to always be truly and fully WHERE we are and WHO we are. Hence, embracing mindfulness propels us closer to achieving wellness - a state of complete harmony of the body, mind, and soul.

# Chapter 4. Getting Started: Basics of Mindful Eating

Eating. An act as routine as breathing, often subsumed in our daily hustle without much thought. But what if you were told that the way you eat could transform your relationship with food, enhancing not only your physical health but mental wellbeing too? Welcome to the world of Mindful Eating - a practice deeply rooted in the concept of mindfulness. But before we dive deep, let's first grasp its fundamental tenets.

## 4.1. Understanding Mindful Eating

Mindful eating is, at its core, about being fully present for the experience of eating, paying close attention to the sensations, thoughts, and emotions that arise during a meal or snack. As opposed to the unconscious, rushed, and often mechanical act of eating many of us are accustomed to, mindful eating instills a profound sense of respect and gratitude towards food and your body.

## 4.2. Why Mindful Eating

Mindful eating can reduce overeating and bingeing, help you tune into your body's unique nutritional needs, assist with weight management, and savour the pleasure of eating. It also contributes to better digestion, as eating mindfully supports slower, more thorough chewing, and less overall food intake. It cultivates a healthy attitude toward food and body, liberating you from destructive dieting patterns and food guilt.

# 4.3. The Roots: Mindfulness

However, we must recognize that mindful eating is a mere extension of the wider mindfulness practice. Deriving its origins from Buddhist teachings, mindfulness is the practice of being wholly present, heightening our awareness of both internal and external environments without judgment. It provides you with the tools to gains insight into your thoughts, emotions, and behaviours inherent in your relationship with food.

# 4.4. The Pillars of Mindful Eating

1. **Mindful Check-in** – Before you start eating, take a moment to assess your hunger and fullness levels. Pay attention to physical hunger and satiety cues instead of eating based on time, emotions or external cues.

2. **Sensation Awareness** – Notice the colours, aroma, textures, and flavours of your food. Savour each bite, grounding yourself in the sensory experience.

3. **Mindful Swallowing** – Consciously notice the process of chewing and swallowing. Eating slowly promotes better digestion.

4. **Non-Judgment** – Cultivate an attitude of non-judgment towards yourself and your food. Release guilt, shame or anxieties associated with eating.

5. **Mindful Resilience** – Accept that there will be mindful meals and mindless ones. Develop resilience to move past the mindless meals without discouragement or guilt.

# 4.5. Embarking on a Mindful Eating Journey

Embracing mindful eating isn't about overnight successes or quick fixes. It's a journey of self-discovery and patience. To get started, let's break it down into manageable steps.

1. **Start small** - Begin with one meal or snack each day, gradually building up to more meals.

2. **Create a conducive environment** - Designate a quiet, comfortable place for mindful meals. Remove distractions like phones, TV, and work materials.

3. **Tune In** - Check in with your feelings of hunger and fullness before, during and after meals. Note the emotions that surface, without judgment.

4. **Slow Down** - Aim to chew each mouthful of food around 20-30 times before swallowing. This will help you savor your food, aid digestion, and make you fuller sooner.

5. **Appreciate your food** - Before each meal, take a moment to appreciate the effort that went into the preparation of your food. This helps cultivate gratitude, making your meal more satisfying.

# 4.6. Common Challenges and Strategies

Just like any new practice, mindful eating can come with its own set of challenges. Let's address these roadblocks and arm ourselves with suitable strategies.

1. **Distractions** - It's easy to get distracted during meals. In such cases, remind yourself gently and bring your focus back to the food.

2. **Automatic Eating** - We're often so conditioned to eating that it becomes an automatic act. With patience, persist with the practice of mindful eating until it integrates into your routine.

3. **Feeling of Deprivation** - Initially, you might feel deprived,

especially if you are reducing your meal portions or giving up comfort foods. Recognize these feelings, provide self-compassion, and remind yourself of your goal towards mindful eating.

Don't gauge your journey by the number of perfect mindful meals. Instead, appreciate each new insight, knowledge, and resilience you develop along the way: That is the true essence of the mindful eating journey.

Let this be not only the start of a new chapter in your nutritional habits but a more mindful and balanced lifestyle. Immerse yourself in the flavors of mindfulness; remember, it's less about the destination and more about a flavorful journey. So let's embark on this enriching voyage, one bite at a time.

# Chapter 5. Harmonizing Fitness Routines with Mindfulness Techniques

Fitness, a vital part of holistic wellbeing, is as much about the body as it is about the mind. As you journey through the practice of incorporating mindfulness into your fitness routine, it's important to remember that mindfulness, while a distinct practice, can beautifully harmonize with your fitness schedule, thereby enhancing the benefits. This section unravels this symbiosis between mindfulness and fitness, and guides you to transform your regular workout routine into a mindful one.

## 5.1. Attuning to the Here and Now

Mindfulness at its core is about being "in the moment." In the fitness context, this means paying acute attention to your body, the exercises, your breathing patterns, and even the sweat trickling down your forehead. Practicing fitness with an autopilot mindset often results in mundane and ineffective routines, while mindfulness inculcates an openness to new experiences.

To attune yourself to the here and now, begin by tuning into your senses. As you perform each exercise, notice how your muscles tense and relax. Try to discern individual muscular movements instead of lumping it all as 'exercising.' Pay equal attention to your breathing. Is it synchronized with your movements? If not, can you harmonize them?

# 5.2. Creating Mindful Fitness Routines

Below are some ways you can ingrain mindfulness in your fitness routines.

1. **Slow down**: Speed often eclipses mindfulness. By slowing your pace, you create the mental space to observe your movement patterns and acknowledge the work put in by different body parts.

2. **Tune in to your body**: Each body speaks a unique language. Understanding this language helps gauge when to push harder and when to ease. Pay attention to how your body responds to different postures and exercises.

3. **Focus on breathing**: Conscious breathing bridges the gap between body and mind. It is a tangible part of exercise that you can direct and regulate even while managing complex physical activities.

# 5.3. The Importance of Mindful Warm-ups

Warm-ups prepare your body for the impending physical workout. But they can also aid in preparing your mind. By focusing on each muscle as you warm up, you can activate your body and mind simultaneously. This is an opportunity not just to prepare your muscles for what's coming but also to remind your mind to stay present throughout.

It is beneficial to take a couple of minutes before starting your workout to ground yourself. Close your eyes, start taking deep inhalations and exhalations, and slowly open your eyes maintaining this slow, deep breath pattern.

# 5.4. Connecting Fitness with Breath

Breathing exercises, or Pranayama, are a core tenet of yoga that can seamlessly blend with any exercise routine. Mastering your breath can multiply the benefits of fitness, mainly by improving oxygenation, developing better control over the body, and calming the mind.

Here's how you can implement it:

1. **Running and jogging**: Match your strides with breaths. Inhale for four strides and exhale for the next four.

2. **Weightlifting**: Exhale when you exert force (lifting) and inhale when you relax (lowering).

3. **Yoga**: Each asana is coupled with specific instructions for inhalation and exhalation. Follow the instructions closely.

# 5.5. Embracing the Silence

As the world around you wakes up, embrace the silence inside of you. Early morning workouts, particularly, can provide the quiet surroundings for a peaceful fitness routine. However, if mornings don't work for you, find other quiet pockets in your day.

# 5.6. Learning from Setbacks

Nobody is perfect. There will be days when you falter or might not be able to work out with the intended intensity. Instead of viewing it as a failure, perceive it as a learning opportunity, a moment to understand your limitations and expand your boundaries.

Embedding mindfulness into your workout regimen nurtures not just a fit body but also a tranquil mind. It can convert a mechanical process into one that promotes growth and learning. As you move along this path, remember that the journey matters just as much as the destination. Our next section will explore mindful eating and how to achieve nutritional balance.

# Chapter 6. Cultivating a Mindful Relationship with Food: Strategies and Techniques

With an improved awareness of how our bodies and minds respond to the food we eat, we become more capable of making discerning, healthy choices, not out of responsibility or obligation but out of genuine care and respect for our well-being.

## 6.1. Understanding Mindful Eating

Mindful eating is based on mindfulness, a form of meditation that helps you recognize and cope with your emotions and physical sensations. It's about tuning in rather than tuning out while you eat. It involves enjoying your food by engaging all the senses, acknowledging your responses to food (likes, dislikes, or neutral), learning to be aware of physical hunger and satiety cues to guide decision-making about when to begin and end eating, and being aware of and challenging your responses to food-related cues to prevent overeating.

## 6.2. The Impact of Mindless Eating

To put mindful eating into perspective, let's first look at its converse - mindless eating. This is a state where we eat without paying attention to what, how much, and the quality of what we're eating.

Mindless eating can lead to overeating, emotional eating, or eating out of boredom. Over time, such habits can escalate into more adverse health effects such as obesity, diabetes, heart diseases, etc.

# Chapter 7. The Art Of Savoring Your Meal

The act of eating is often reduced to a task or a hurried process in our fast-paced world. However, savoring a meal is an essential facet of mindful eating. Here are some techniques:

1. Slow down your eating pace: Chew thoroughly to ease digestion and absorb more nutrients.

2. Engage your senses: Observe the color, texture, and aroma of the food before eating.

3. Minimize distractions: Avoid screens or reading during mealtime. Be present.

4. Acknowledge your food: Consider the effort it took to produce and cook your meal.

# 7.1. Techniques to Cultivate Mindful Eating

There are several beneficial techniques that you can adopt to improve your relationship with food.

1. Practice Hunger Awareness: Recognize your body's hunger cues. Before eating, ask yourself if you're eating out of hunger or for other reasons.

2. Tune into Fullness: It's just as important to recognize when you're satiated as when you're hungry.

3. Non-Judgment: If you have eaten past fullness, simply note it and plan to pause halfway through the next meal to check in with yourself about how full you are.

4. Be Mindful of Emotional Eating: Becoming aware of triggers for

emotional eating and finding other ways to feed your feelings.

## 7.2. Incorporating Mindful Eating into Your Daily Routine

Bringing mindfulness to your dining table doesn't have to be a daunting task. Start with small steps and gradually incorporate more practices.

**Start with one meal a day: Begin with one meal, possibly breakfast when you're less likely to be rushed.**

**Take small bites and chew thoroughly:** This helps digestion and gives your brain the necessary time to recognize when your body is full.

# Be grateful: Before you begin a meal, take a moment to feel gratitude for your food — for the nourishment it offers, for the people who produced it, and for the privilege of having food on your table.

Through consistent practice, mindful eating can become a powerful tool to regain control of your nutritional health. Stay patient and persistent for mental transformations take time but are usually resilient.

## .1. Treating Food as Nourishment

One of the fundamental changes in cultivating mindful eating is to start viewing food as nourishment and not just as a source of pleasure or a solution for boredom. Begin to consider the quality of food you consume—the rich micronutrients, the source of your food, how it fuels and empowers your body, how it heals, and strengthens you.

To reiterate, the idea is not about being stringent but being cognizant, not about dieting or eliminating favorite foods but about balance and making informed decisions.

# .2. Conclusion: Cultivate and Nourish

Mindful eating is an effective strategy for maintaining a healthy relationship with food. It encourages a holistic view of food, one that recognizes and respects the interplay of mind, body, and food. By turning mindful attention to the food you eat, you imbue everyday routines with greater meaning and transform the necessary into a delightful ritual of self-care and wellness. So, explore the principles of mindful eating and nourish both your body and soul with conscious engagement.

# Chapter 8. Combating Stress & Anxiety: Mindfulness as your Ally

As our investigation into mindfulness and its impact on wellness deepens, we will now turn our attention to the enormous task of managing stress and anxiety, pervasive issues that can profoundly affect our physical health, our mental balance, and our overall satisfaction with life. With the aid of mindfulness, we can learn to navigate these tumultuous waters with greater ease, leading to an improved state of wellbeing.

## 8.1. Understanding Stress and Anxiety

Before we can address stress and anxiety, it's crucial that we fully comprehend what these concepts mean. Stress, in essence, is our body's response to perceived threats or challenges. This may include imminent dangers (such as avoiding an oncoming car) or more abstract matters like work deadlines or interpersonal conflicts. In response to these perceived threats, our body initiates a "fight or flight" reaction, releasing hormones like adrenaline and cortisol that heighten our senses, quicken our pulse, and prepare our bodies to respond.

Anxiety, on the other hand, extends slightly beyond the immediate responses encompassed by stress. It's an uneasy feeling of fear or apprehension that often persists even when the source of worry is unclear, and it may be constant and overwhelming, markedly reducing our quality of life.

Both stress and anxiety, while generally viewed negatively, do serve functions vital to human survival and functioning. However, when these reactions become chronic, it consumes significant energy and can lead to a host of physical and mental health issues, from heart disease and autoimmune disorders to depression and memory difficulties.

# 8.2. The Power of Mindfulness: Observing without Judging

Fortunately, this is where mindfulness enters the scene. Mindfulness involves bringing one's attention to experiences happening in the present moment, without judgment. When practicing mindfulness, you're not aiming to change anxious thoughts and feelings, but to develop a new relationship with them- a relationship where they have less influence over you.

To put it simply, the power of mindfulness lies in its ability to help us step back and observe our experiences, rather than getting caught up in them. When we experience a thought or feeling that typically triggers stress or anxiety, mindful observation allows us to recognize the thought or feeling for what it is: a temporary, passing experience, not a fixed aspect of our self or our life.

# 8.3. Mindfulness Techniques to Combat Stress and Anxiety

Now that we have a basic understanding of how mindfulness can help us manage stress and anxiety let's delve deeper into several valuable mindfulness techniques.

### 8.3.1. Mindfulness-Based Stress Reduction (MBSR)

MBSR is a program that assists people in learning how to calm their minds and bodies to help them cope with stress, pain, and illness. It involves a mix of mindfulness meditation, body awareness, and yoga, and participants are encouraged to practice these skills in their daily lives.

## 8.3.2. Mindful Breathing

This involves concentrating on your breath, observing each inhalation and exhalation, and acknowledging your thoughts as they come and go. Observing your breath diverts your mind away from the worries that are fuelling your anxiety. It's a simple exercise that you can do virtually anywhere.

## 8.3.3. Body Scan

This meditation encourages individuals to check in with their bodies and actually experience the physical sensations that often go unnoticed. Starting from the toes and moving upward, you bring awareness to each part of the body, observing without judgment.

# 8.4. Integrating Mindfulness into Everyday Life

The best part about mindfulness is that it can be integrated into your everyday routine without requiring large stretches of time. Here are a few suggestions:

## 8.4.1. Mindful Eating

Rather than consuming meals mindlessly while watching television or working, take this time to truly experience your food. Take note of the textures, flavors, colors, smells, and even the sounds your food makes. Put your utensils down between bites, and chew thoroughly. This practice isn't just beneficial for stress and anxiety; it can also improve digestion and our relationship with food.

## 8.4.2. Mindful Walking

Pay attention to the contact of your feet with the ground, the sway of your arms as they move, the breeze against your face, and the sounds around you. Walking, a routine act, can become a source of deep presence and calmness.

## 8.4.3. Mindful Pauses

Consider setting alarms or reminders throughout the day to engage in one-minute mindful pauses. During these pauses, pay attention to your breath, your physical sensations, and the sounds around you. Recognize any thoughts or worries that are present, and enable them to pass without judgment.

# 8.5. A Lifestyle Shift

Addressing stress and anxiety with mindfulness doesn't mean your life will suddenly become free of worry or tension- that is not the goal. It's about recognizing and embracing these experiences as a part of life, yet not letting them have power over you. It's about developing resilience- not resistance- to hardships. Remember, transform doesn't occur overnight. It needs your commitment and patience; it needs your compassion. However, it's a trip worth taking, for it leads us to a destination of balance and wellbeing.

Overcoming stress and anxiety is just one piece of the mindfulness puzzle, but a significant one. As your mindfulness practice deepens, you'll discover more about yourself and how you relate to the world around you, leading to a healthier, more balanced way of life. Now that's too good a treasure to pass up, don't you think?

# Chapter 9. Creating Your Mindful Fitness and Diet Plan: Practical Guidelines

Your transformative journey begins when you set clear objectives and design a plan to meet them. The following practical guidelines will help you create a mindful fitness and nutrition program that's tailored to your current situation and future goals.

## 9.1. Assess Your Baseness, Define Your Goals

Before committing to any fitness or nutritional plan, it's essential to understand your baseline. What's your current level of fitness? How does your daily food intake look? Knowing your starting point will help place your goals in context. You can start by jotting down:

1. Your weight, BMI, and body fat percentage.
2. Your average daily calorie intake.
3. The type of physical activity you currently engage in, if any.

Your goal could be to lose a certain amount of weight, increase strength or flexibility, or simply improve general health. Cultivating mindfulness can help you align your fitness and nutritional aim with your broader well-being objectives.

## 9.2. Creating a Mindful Fitness Plan

Crafting a mindfulness-infused fitness program requires attention and concentration, focusing on what your body is experiencing during physical activity. Start with :

1. *Choose activities you enjoy*: It's easier to stick with activities you like. Whether it's swimming, yoga, running, or group exercises, make sure you love it.

2. *Set manageable schedules*: Be realistic with your time. Always maintain a balance between your routine and your fitness schedule.

3. *Focus on each movement*: Experience the sensation as you move, maintaining mindfulness while exercising helps improve performance, reduces the risk of injury, and enhances enjoyment.

## 9.3. Your Mindful Nutrition Plan

Adopting a mindfully nutritious lifestyle goes beyond counting calories. It's about noticing your body's hunger and satiety cues, understanding your relationship with food, and making mindful decisions.

1. *Eating strategically*: Align your meals with your activities for the day. If you know today is a high-intensity workout day, plan for higher protein intake.

2. *Have a balanced plate*: Make sure your meals are balanced with protein, carbohydrates, and fats. Don't cut out any food groups unless advised by a health professional.

3. *Practice mindful eating*: Savor the food, pay attention to how it makes you feel, notice when you're full. This practice can help control overeating and enhance the pleasure of meals.

## 9.4. Monitoring Your Progress

It is vital to track your progress to maintain momentum and make necessary adjustments. Use an activity tracker, keep a food diary, or use tracking apps. Remember, progress is not linear. There will be ups and downs, but perseverance and mindfulness are critical.

# 9.5. Practicing Mindful Rest

Finally, rest is as crucial as exercise. Sleep and rest are integral to overall well-being and providing your body with recovery time. Practice mindful rest, paying attention to the quality of your sleep, and taking time out for relaxation.

By integrating mindfulness into your fitness and diet plan, you'll not only achieve physical transformations but will also open doors to improved mental well-being. As you progress in your journey, always take stock of how you feel. The ultimate goal is to nourish and strengthen your body while nourishing your mind too. Such a balanced approach will ensure you grow healthier, fitter, and calmer. With persistence, patience, and mindfulness, you'll be on your way to a well-balanced lifestyle.

# Chapter 10. Inspiring Stories - Success Tales from the Realm of Mindful Fitness and Nutrition

It's often said that motivation can be found in the success tales of others, and this holds true for individuals embarking on their respective journeys towards mindful fitness and nutritional balance.

## 10.1. A Full-Circle Revolution: Sam's Sojourn

Sam is a 35-year-old software engineer, who barely had any time to devote to his health due to his demanding job. His hectic schedule left him with an unbalanced diet and no time for exercise. Overweight, constantly tired, and battling precarious health indicators, transforming seemed an impossible task.

However, a chance engagement with a mindfulness workshop made him realize the power of meditation and mindful living. Sam decided to practice mindfulness not just in isolation, but within the confines of his workout and diet as well.

His day started off with mindfulness meditation, followed by a consciously prepared breakfast of whole grains, fruits, and protein. By taking time to savor each bite, Sam became more aware of the quality and quantity of his intake, leading to healthier choices. In the evenings, he combined mindfulness techniques with physical exercises like walking or cycling. This helped him in becoming more attuned with his body during the workout, leading to better accountability and performance.

After six months of this regime, Sam saw transformative results. His weight was healthier, his energy levels had shot up, and his mood had vastly improved. Sam's transformation was a testament to the might of mindfulness, a tale of a well-rounded approach towards fitness and nutrition.

## 10.2. From Weight-loss Woes to Wellness Wins: Sophie's Story

Next, let's delve into Sophie's story, a 28-year-old accountant who was struggling with post-pregnancy weight and a body image crisis. Her initial, rushed attempts at weight loss had not just drained her physically but also mentally due to unrealistic dieting norms and insane fitness schedules.

Stumbling upon a mindfulness seminar, Sophie realized her approach was flawed. She needed to focus not just on losing weight but achieving overall wellness. Thus began her journey towards mindfulness.

Sophie chose mindful eating, which made her understand, enjoy, and control her eating habits better by considering the sensory experiences of the foods she was consuming. Through Yoga and Pilates, Sophie took mindful fitness to heart, appreciating the movements of her body and its resilience.

After a year, Sophie didn't just achieve her weight goal but also developed a fresh perspective towards food and fitness. She was mentally healthier, proving that mindful practices could lead to profound transformations far beyond physical appearances.

## 10.3. Busting the Myth of Age-limit: George's Transformation

George, a 60-year-old retiree, had resigned himself to the idea of a sedentary lifestyle, believing his age hindered him from any fitness pursuits. But when a chance encounter with a marathon runner in his seventies shocked him out of this mindset, he decided to step out of his comfort zone.

George adopted a mindfulness regime, emphasizing gentle yet impactful physical activities like tai-chi, swimming, and even strength training. He paid careful attention to his body's needs as he exercised, thus facilitating an incredibly personal and effective route towards fitness, without overstressing his body. His nutritional plan was well-balanced, and he practiced mindful eating, ensuring adequate nutrition without depriving his palate.

A year later, George surprised everyone, including himself, by running a 5k marathon. His story is an inspiring testament that age does not define our fitness boundaries - our mindset does!

## 10.4. Overcoming the Overwhelm: James and Emotional Eating

James was a 45-year-old investment banker under constant stress, resulting in emotional eating. His unhealthy relationship with food was creating mental and physical chaos, making him an image of the paradox of modern life – materially affluent but health bankrupt.

A nutritional wellness seminar introduced James to mindfulness. He started practicing mindful eating which led him towards understanding his emotional triggers and how to manage them better. He began fitness routines where he took time to focus on every movement, every breath, synchronizing his mind and body.

What followed was a miraculous transformation. Six months later, James was not just physically healthier, but his quality of life had improved leaps and bounds. By identifying, addressing, and managing his food-related emotions, he'd balanced his nutritional intake as a whole, thereby redefining his approach towards health and wellness.

In conclusion, these stories underline the power of transforming through mindfulness. By integrating mindfulness in fitness and nutritional plans, these individuals turned their health around, both physically and mentally. They serve as inspirations for us, reinforcing the effectiveness of mindfulness in achieving well-rounded health outcomes. By immersing in this process mindfully, we establish a wholesome connection with ourselves, understanding and respecting our bodies' needs and nourishing them as required - the very essence of mindful fitness and nutritional balance.

# Chapter 11. Overcoming Obstacles on the Path to Mindful Fitness and Nutrition

As with any wellness journey, traversing the path towards mindful fitness and nutrition is not without its hurdles. Overcoming these obstacles is an inherent part of the voyage, propelling personal growth, solidifying dedication, and teaching invaluable lessons about oneself.

## 11.1. Identifying Challenges on the Path

The initial step towards overcoming hurdles is identifying what these challenges might be. Are they related to time management? Perhaps lack of knowledge or skills? Or, are they rooted in mental barriers like motivation, self-esteem, or stress?

Some common obstacles to mindful fitness and nutrition include:

- **Lack of Time:** In the fast-paced rhythm of life, finding time for exercise and meal planning can be challenging.

- **Limited Knowledge/Understanding:** Understanding the finer details of fitness and nutrition can seem daunting and discouraging for newcomers. Information overload is real and every source seems to propose a "best" diet or exercise routine.

- **Motivation:** Maintaining consistency in one's fitness and nutrition journey can feel laborious without appropriate motivation.

- **Physical Limitations:** Injuries or certain health conditions may restrict the ability to engage in certain exercises.

- **Mental Health Barriers:** Stress, low self-esteem, or psychological conditions can thwart fitness and nutrition efforts.

## 11.2. Tackling Time Constraints

Time can be one of the biggest hinderances to maintaining fitness and nutrition, but with mindfulness, we can control our schedules rather than being governed by them. Here are some suggestions:

- **Prioritize:** Just as you would pencil in a business meeting into your schedule, so should you mark personal workout or meal planning. Make these non-negotiable appointments with yourself.

- **Combine Activities:** Evaluate your day and see where you can combine activities or multitask. Listen to an enlightening podcast while cooking. Use your lunch break to take a brisk walk.

- **Micro-Workouts:** If carving out a full hour feels overwhelming, try slotting in smaller, more intense workouts throughout the day.

## 11.3. Overcoming Knowledge Deficits

Starting a fitness and nutrition regimen without prior knowledge can be daunting but certainly not insurmountable. Here are ways to conquer this impediment:

- **Educate Yourself:** Start by learning the basics of nutrition and fitness. Nutrition books, online blogs, documentaries, or professional health and fitness courses can all be vast sources of knowledge.

- **Find a Mentor:** Find a fitness trainer or a nutritionist who can guide you. They can customize a routine based on your personal needs and provide valuable insights.

- **Team Up:** Join a fitness group or nutrition club. Shared knowledge can help you learn faster.

# 11.4. Igniting Motivation

Motivation is a complex issue and lacks a one-size-fits-all solution. It requires mindful and constant efforts:

- **Find Your 'Why':** Your 'why' is the core reason you want to adopt a fitness and nutrition regimen. It could be health, aesthetics, or personal improvement. Use this 'why' as your guiding light in moments of wavering motivation.

- **Set SMART goals:** Goals should be Specific, Measurable, Achievable, Relevant, and Time-bound. These help monitor progress and stay motivated.

- **Celebrate Small Victories:** The path towards mindfulness is a marathon, not a sprint. Celebrate the small victories along the way to keep motivation high.

# 11.5. Dealing with Physical Limitations

Physical limitations can seem daunting but can be tackled wisely:

- **Individualized Exercise Routine:** Consult with a physical therapist or fitness expert. Let them design an exercise routine that suits your physical capabilities.

- **Alternative Activities:** Engage in lower-impact exercises like yoga, swimming, or Pilates. They can be less strenuous while still providing health benefits.

- **Patience Is Key:** Healing takes time. Don't rush the process or force your body to perform beyond its current capabilities.

# 11.6. Overcoming Mental Health Barriers

Mental health and wellness are fundamentally linked. If mental health becomes a barrier, consider these methods:

- **Mindful Practices:** Incorporating mindfulness practices like meditation, deep breathing, or self-reflection can enhance mental well-being.

- **Counseling:** Mental health professionals can provide tools necessary to combat stress, low self-esteem, anxiety, or depressive symptoms.

- **Positive Affirmation:** Constant self-reminders of personal strength, worth, and courage can fortify your resolve against mental health hurdles.

Obstacles are part of every journey, but when viewed through the lens of mindfulness, they become opportunities for personal growth. On your path towards a mindful lifestyle, be kind, patient, and forgiving towards yourself. Remember, it's not about perfection but progression. View every setback as a stepping stone towards a healthier, more mindful you.

# Chapter 12. Future Scope: Mindfulness, Fitness, and Nutrition in a Changing World

The winds of change have swept across every realm of human existence, leaving no stone unturned - including our perspectives towards fitness and nutrition. The future holds an amalgamation of mindful living, vitality-enhancing fitness regimens, and nutrition-conscious choices, all enveloped in the warmth of sustainable practices.

## 12.1. The New Fitness Paradigm

Fitness in the future pertains not only to the physical, but the holistic state of well-being. The age-old belief of 'Exercise to Burn Calories' will progressively transform into 'Exercise to Boost Mental and Emotional Health.'

As global technological advancements take the spotlight, the role of virtual and augmented reality in transforming our fitness routines will be significant. They'll help simulate outdoor fitness experiences within our homes, increasing convenience without compromising on the 'fun' factor. Fitness trackers and wearables will further escalate in their capabilities, providing us with intricate insights about our health and helping us customize our fitness regimes to suit our unique needs.

The concept of gamification will make fitness excitingly engaging, making the journey to health less rigorous and more enjoyable. We'll see a rise in competitive fitness gaming and collaborative online workout sessions, bridging geographical boundaries and fostering relationships through our shared wellness journeys.

## 12.2. Mindfulness: The Lynchpin of Holistic Health

As we dive deeper into the future, mindfulness will no longer be considered an optional practice but an integral aspect of our overall well-being.

Mindfulness, being the art of being fully present, will help individuals combat the psychological implications of incessantly busy, digitally driven lives. It will be infused into every activity, from doing household chores to doing professional tasks, making everything a process of conscious living.

Further, the application of mindfulness in fitness will gain traction, nurturing mind-body harmony. Activities like Yoga and Tai Chi, that practice mindful movement, will see a surge, as they provide a grounding experience that modern fast-paced workouts may not offer. Mindful Eating, paying full attention to our food intake process, will also soar in popularity, addressing issues like binge-eating and unhealthy diet patterns.

## 12.3. Nutrition: More than just Food Intake

In the future, the nutrition sphere will extend beyond just supplying our bodies with energy to providing nourishment at a cellular level, enhancing the overall functioning of the system.

Personalized nutrition will be the show stopper. Genetic, epigenetic, and microbiotic testing will help design diet plans curated explicitly for individuals, countering the 'one-size-fits-all' approach.

Sustainability will also be a crucial aspect of our nutritional choices. The burgeoning demand for plant-based and lab-grown meat options signifies a shift towards embracing approaches that are not just beneficiary for our health, but also kind to our planet.

# 12.4. Reimagining the Healthcare Space

The future will witness a crossover of healthcare with mindfulness, fitness, and nutrition, ensuing a shift from disease-centric approaches to prevention-centric ones.

Use of telemedicine and technology based diagnostic tools will surge, making healthcare more accessible and efficient. Further, mental health will take center stage alongside physical health, underscoring the need for balance between both for leading a healthier life.

Healthcare providers will increasingly leverage mindfulness techniques, nutrition counseling, and activity-based therapy as part of primary care. Health insurance will also be revolutionized - risk assessments will not be limited to age and hereditary factors; instead, they will incorporate fitness habits, nutrition preferences, and how integrally mindfulness is practiced by the insured.

The future, though unpredictable, seems promising. It offers us a renewed perspective - one that perceives fitness, nutrition, and mindfulness, not as separate entities, but as interconnected threads of the same fabric - our wellbeing. With this understanding, let each one of us contribute, evolve, and tread together on the path of creating this harmonious world.

www.ingramcontent.com/pod-product-compliance
Lightning Source LLC
Chambersburg PA
CBHW071010260726
48661CB00007B/2878